A HANDBOOK ON CARING FOR SOMEONE WITH CANCER

Instructions for the Support Person or Caregiver Helping a Loved One Survive Cancer

Written By

Teryn Jones

Copyright

ISBN: 979-8-49698-071-5

Table of Contents

PREFACE

My guess is that you have chosen to read this book because you know and want to help someone who has been diagnosed with cancer. My intention in writing this book is to share some of the knowledge I acquired on my journey as a support person, and hopefully this information will provide you with somewhat of a roadmap that will help your journey go smoothly. For the purpose of providing gender neutrality, the words 'they' or 'the patient' will often be used in this book instead of 'him' or 'her'.

This handbook will guide you through the process of how to support someone who is being challenged with the diagnosis of cancer, its treatments and hopefully their road to recovery. Not all types of cancer can be cured. For the purposes of this handbook, the incurable cancers are considered an adjacent topic that also require coping with different levels of detachment. The goal here is to help a loved one get through surviving cancer, and for this reason the management of a terminal illness and/or the need for hospice will not be addressed.

Ultimately, it's hard to know what to do or say when someone tells you they have cancer. I hope this book can help you understand how a cancer patient might feel. Your understanding of their mindset and emotions will help you to be a better support person during their time of need.

1. I FOUND OUT MY FRIEND HAD CANCER

Our journey began with an ordinary call, on an ordinary day, from one of my closest friends. We usually spoke daily, so there was nothing alarming or unexpected about seeing her name when my cell phone rang so early that morning.

"Hey, good morning!" I said as I often did on our first call of the day.

We generally checked in with each other sometime during the morning on most days. We'd call each other just to chat about a television show, to gripe about work or even something as simple as the weather. We never needed a reason to call, we routinely called each other because that was the standard with our friendship.

"Good morning, how are you?" She replied, but I could tell by the melancholy tone of her voice that something was a little off with her.

"Are you okay?" I asked.

"Well," she started right in, "I found a lump in my breast when I was doing a self-exam this morning."

I was a little dumbfounded at the information and didn't immediately know how to respond. I had to take a few seconds to mentally digest her words.

"Did you hear me?" She asked.

"Yeah, yeah, I was just thinking about it" I responded while still trying to pull the words together for a real response. I followed that with, "I'm sure it's nothing to worry about. It's probably some fat tissue or something that you just hadn't noticed before." That was the best I could come up with in trying not to sound alarmed. Plus, I sort of believed what I was saying because no one close to me had ever had Breast Cancer.

"You're probably right, except it's disturbing because I just had a mammogram two months ago and it was negative, so I think I'm going to make an appointment with my doctor to have it checked out, just in case." We both agreed that a doctor's visit was probably the most sensible action in order for us to rule out the "C" word... cancer.

Since the lump was found only a few short months after her mammogram, the doctor rushed my friend in for another mammogram. It only took a couple of days for the doctor to call with the results, and unfortunately it was bad news; the results showed a tumor in her breast. The next step was for her return to the doctor for a biopsy of the tumor to determine if it was benign or malignant. A malignant tumor would mean it was cancerous.

My friend was an independent woman. She had served in the military, put herself through college, and was doing an incredible job of raising her daughter as a single parent. But as one can imagine, the threat of a potential diagnosis that may end with death, is not information someone might want to receive alone. She asked me to go to the doctor with her. Fortunately, I was able to arrange my work schedule and we met at the doctor's office. If the news was going to be good or bad, I wanted to be there to rejoice or cry with her. Within days we were back sitting in the doctor's office awaiting the results of the biopsy. When the doctor came in, he greeted us both and got right down to the facts without mixing further pleasantries. Her worst fear was confirmed. We could not rule out the big "C". She had Breast Cancer.

Finding out that my friend had Breast Cancer was not only traumatizing for her, but for me as well. My first thought was: "how can I support her through this?" I impulsively told her that she could count on me to be there for whatever she needed, but in hindsight, and in all honesty, I should not have voiced my intentions until I'd had a chance to listen and understand the expectations and challenges of a support person. Being a support person to a friend or loved one may be a choice, or it might be more of a necessity because you are the closest person to give this service. If possible, it will be wiser and much smarter to first obtain some knowledge about the demands and assistances cancer requires from both the patient and support person, before you commit your time, energy and performance.

During my adult life, I've never had a loved one or close friend who was diagnosed with cancer, so I was completely unprepared for the mental, physical and emotional exhaustion that came with caring for someone with cancer. Now, with that being said, I wouldn't change a single thing; however, it would've been nice to have a 'head's-up' of what I was agreeing to before saying 'I'll be there for whatever you need'.

I will admit that my journey as a cancer support person was not in any way equal or similar to my friend's cancer journey, and I'll further state that her experience was probably five to ten times worse than mine, but what I'm trying to respectfully communicate is that this was a difficult journey for both of us.

I am not a doctor or nurse, nor am I employed in any other position related to the medical profession. I am just a person who deeply cared for a friend with cancer. I volunteered to be her support person. This is not a decision that I regret in any way and I would gladly do it again. However, the reason I'd accept the responsibility again is because I now know what to expect. It is a big undertaking that comes with challenges and accomplishments.

As a support person, it is important to know that there will be times when everything goes according to plan and your days are flowing like a well-oiled machine. These will be the moments to smile and rejoice at the small triumphs and the big milestones. Yet, it is equally important to know that there will be far more times when you feel helpless and unable to help with their pain and discomfort. These are the times that will require a great deal of your patience, compassion, and physical or emotional energy, along with the acceptance of what you can and can't do.

2. CANCER

When someone has told you they have cancer, it's common to not know what to say or do. For me, my first response was with thoughts of fear. What did this mean? Was she going to die? Could she recover? There are so many unknowns and unanswered questions that come with a cancer diagnosis; it's completely reasonable to become speechless or either have feelings of anger, resentment or shock when the news is received.

Your loved one has shared their cancer diagnosis with you because you're someone they trust to be caring and compassionate towards their plight. Neither of you knows exactly how this will change your lives, but what you already may know and I can also tell you is that cancer is a horrible disease that attacks targeted cells in the body; it changes their function and uncontrollably spreads to surrounding cells, tissues, organs and other parts of the body. It can eventually kill its host unless treatment to fight it is aggressive and successful.

Now let's talk about cancer. Cancer is a malignancy, which means that the cancer cells will divide abnormally and uncontrollably while destroying the body tissues around them. The cancerous cells usually form into a tumor that will attempt to also spread into surrounding areas. The cells can also invade the immune system and spread through the body's lymphatic and circulatory networks.

Oncology is the branch of medicine that treats cancer. The oncology staff assigned to a cancer patient will typically include the Oncologist, which is the doctor that treats the cancer, a Registered Oncology Nurse who specializes in care and education for cancer patients, and an Oncology Social Worker. The Social Worker can help the patient and you as the support person, with counseling needs, support groups, transportation, financial resources and an array of other practical services.

It has been said that cancer infects more than ten million people around the globe each year. Some of it grows and spreads fast, and other types may spread slow and over several years.

Cancer can start in almost any part of the body. Most major concerns are with the fast-growing cancers. Some of the more common and fastest growing cancers include the following:

Leukemia: this cancer attacks the bone marrow and spreads its disease by suppressing the production of normal blood cells.

Breast Cancers: These cancers can occur in both women and men; however, they are more common in women. The two most aggressive types are:

Inflammatory Breast Cancer, in which case the cancer cells spread in the vessels of the immune system that covers the breasts. With this type of cancer, the breast may appear red or swollen.

The second most aggressive type of Breast Cancer is Triple Negative Breast Cancer. This one isn't as easy to visually detect as the Inflammatory Breast Cancer. It's called Triple Negative because the cancer cells do not have estrogen receptors, nor progesterone receptors, nor much of a protein called HER2, and the spread of these cancer cells cause an excessive hormone imbalance. Self-breast exams, or mammogram screenings may help in detecting early signs of Breast Cancer.

And then there's Lung Cancer. This is a cancer that begins in the lungs and usually, but not always, results from excessive smoking or long time exposure to secondhand smoke. On rare occasion, there may be a family history of Lung Cancer. This type of cancer has symptoms that are sometimes recognizable. The person may have a constant cough or continual wheezing that won't fully go away, or they may complain of continual chest pain. Although this cancer begins in the lungs, it may spread to other parts of the body.

Another fast spreading cancer is Pancreatic Cancer. When cancer starts in the pancreas, it's usually detected late in the disease's progression, because there are no symptoms in its early stages. This is unfortunate because of its ability to spread quickly.

The last cancer I will add to this list of fast growing and fast spreading cancers is Liver Cancer. Like Pancreatic Cancer, there are no obvious symptoms in the early stages, which is why it can go undetected and spread so fast. However, there are subtle differences between the two. In the latter stages of Pancreatic Cancer, the patient may suffer with abdominal pains or frequent vomiting or even begin to have a yellowish skin color. Liver Cancer is generally caused by birth defects, alcohol abuse, or a chronic infection such as Hepatitis B or C.

Some of the slower growing cancers are called Carcinoid Tumors. They can rise in several organs of the body but are usually found in the stomach, the appendix, the small intestine, the colon or the rectum. Cancer in these areas don't generally show symptoms until late in the infection. A common symptom with the Carcinoid Tumors is diarrhea.

One of the most common types of cancer for men is Prostate Cancer. Unlike the other named cancers, this cancer grows very slowly and has few symptoms. Signs that may be associated with this cancer are complaints of difficulty or pain when urinating.

When your loved one tells you they have cancer, more than likely, they will also tell you the type of cancer they have. If it is a cancer that is unfamiliar to you, or even if it is a cancer you've heard of, I would highly urge you to research and learn about the specifics of the cancer. This will help you to understand how it might affect your loved one and their ability to handle the stress, discomforts and changes they'll possibly experience.

Undoubtedly, the biggest question on everyone's mind when they find out that they have cancer is: "Is it curable?"

THE STAGES OF CANCER

When cancer is diagnosed and then confirmed, the doctor will have a conference with the patient and his support person or team to discuss the type and stage of the cancer. This discussion will give details about the size of the tumor (if there is one), its growth pattern and the doctor's suggestions for treatment. However, not all cancers have stages and tumors. For instance, Leukemia doesn't have a stage because it originates in the blood and spreads by changing the blood cells and blood count in various organs.

For the cancers that have stages, there are five characteristic stages and the severity of the cancer gets worse as the number associated with the stage gets higher.

- Stage 0 – Stage zero cancer is when there is a gathering of abnormal cells. The cells are not cancerous at the time of detection, but if not treated, they have the potential of becoming a cancer.

- Stage 1 – Stage one cancer is an early detection of the illness, usually through testing, and typically means the cancer is in one area, has not yet spread, and it can be removed.

- Stage 2 – Stage two cancer means that the cancer has begun to grow and spread, but there's a strong probability that it can still be removed.

- Stage 3 – Stage three cancer is very similar to stage two. But, the cancer is a little larger, though it's still limited to a small area with the possibility that it can be removed.

- Stage 4 – Stage four cancer means the cancer has spread to other areas of the body and most likely cannot be removed. The doctor will possibly attempt treatments that will slow or stop continued spread of the disease.

When someone is diagnosed with a cancer that is staged between zero and three, there is a reasonable chance it will be successfully cured with intensive treatments, and they may still live a long and rewarding life.

Unfortunately, there are others whose diagnosis is found very late in the disease and the cancer has already reached stage four and has uncontrollably spread to other areas of the body. For these persons, the disease is considered incurable.

Finding out cancer has invaded your loved one's body, either curable or incurable, or just knowing they have it is always frightening and alarming. This kind of news is shocking, to say the least. Most people will need to know someone is there for them -- someone they can depend on to help them physically, mentally, emotionally and (if religious) even spiritually when they need it.

Regardless of their personal or mental strengths, the cancer journey is one that very few people will choose to travel alone. Some people are proud and don't want to ask for help, but that doesn't mean they don't need it. You will honor them if you can give them your full attention when you are in their presence and offer your assistance even if it's not requested.

3. THE DIAGNOSIS

The diagnosis is cancer, but what kind? There is literally a cancer that can affect almost every part of the body depending on your age, gender or even ethnicity. There are too many variations of cancers to discuss in this guidebook, so I'm just going to tell you about the ten most common types and how they are sometimes recognized.

I'll start with Skin Cancer. This form of cancer affects more than one million Americans every year. Alarming signs of Skin Cancer might be scaly or red patches on the skin's surface, sores that won't go away or heal, pale or discolored splotches on the skin, wart like growths or sores that may itch or bleed. Skin Cancers tend to form on areas that are continually exposed to ultraviolet (UV) rays, specifically those that come from direct sunlight or tanning beds.

Lung Cancer is another of the most common types of cancer. The symptoms include a persistent cough that worsens over time, chest pain, coughing up blood, hoarseness or a voice change, loss of appetite, wheezing or a shortness of breath. The greatest risk of developing Lung Cancer occurs in cigarette smokers or secondhand smokers. Secondhand smokers are those that are continually in the presence of people who are smoking cigarettes. Although, people who have never smoked can also fall prey to Lung Cancer.

Another common cancer is Prostate Cancer; however, this cancer primarily affects men. This cancer develops in the prostate organ of the male reproductive system. A few of the indicators of a developing tumor may be pain when urinating or reduction of the urine flow to a slow trickling stream, the constant need to urinate, blood in the urine or semen, or erectile dysfunction. Although there are no definite or absolute factors that can be attributed to Prostate Cancer, some doctors have connected prostate inflammation, excessive weight, diet, height and age to all be contributing factors.

One of the leading cancers that primarily affect women is Endometrial Cancer. This cancer invades the endometrial cells of the female uterus. The symptoms may include excessive bleeding between menstrual periods or after menopause. Abnormal vaginal discharge or consistent pelvic pain may also present symptoms. Additional influences of Endometrial Cancer could include an imbalance in the female hormones or undertaking hormone therapy. Endometrial Cancer most often occurs in women after menopause, and they become more at risk for developing this cancer as their age increases.

Breast Cancer is the second most common cancer diagnosed in women; however, it doesn't only affect females. Men do not have breasts, but they have breast tissue and about one percent of diagnosed Breast Cancer occurs in men. There may be a reason to see a doctor if a new lump is detected under the armpit or around the collarbone, if a part of the breast is swollen, if there's peeling or flaking on the breast's surface, or if there's discharge from a nipple. The risk of getting Breast Cancer increases with age and especially in women.

Most Breast Cancer is found in women over the age of fifty, though there are cases where teenagers and young adults have also suffered from Breast Cancer. There are several factors that are associated with Breast Cancer, though a family history of Breast Cancer is thought to be one of the major factors. Also, women with severe obesity, or women who have either had their first pregnancy or a childbirth late in life are likewise at risk for developing this cancer.

Colorectal Cancer is cancer of the colon and rectal areas and it too is one of the leading types of fast-growing cancers. This type of cancer doesn't discriminate and will attack both males and females equally. Most people who are diagnosed with this cancer have usually noticed a drastic change in their bowel movements, but because a person's stool will often change in consistency, they may or may not have been considered it as a serious problem. This change may also be accompanied with abdominal cramping, rectal bleeding, dark brown or black stools, and unintentional weight loss. However, you should be aware that these are not significant signs that only apply to Colorectal Cancer and may also be symptomatic of other colon and bowel problems, such as irritable bowel syndrome or hemorrhoids.

There is no definitive cause of Colorectal Cancer, but some of the associated risks are thought to be diabetes, smoking and excessive alcohol consumption. Other contributors are with persons over fifty years old who have a history of colon polyps or intestinal inflammation. In addition, African Americans tend to have a higher risk of Colorectal Cancer than persons of other races.

Kidney or sometimes called 'Renal' Cancer has been slowly on the rise within the past decade and is now among the top ten cancers in the United States. Men seem to be diagnosed with Kidney Cancer twice as much as women. The possible warning signs of Kidney Cancer are blood in the urine, pain in the lower back that is not the result of an injury, a lump on either side of the lower back, or a persistent fever. A few of the risk factors that are assumed to lead to Kidney Cancer are high blood pressure, obesity, smoking, and like most other cancers the risk increases with age.

Another dreadful offender is Bladder Cancer which usually develops in the inner layers of the bladder and attacks the urinary system. Bladder Cancer can often be detected early because the signs are often painful and not easy to ignore. The patient will most likely have frequent and painful urinations, with the probability of blood in their urine. Little is known about the causes of Bladder Cancer, but it is suspected that tobacco use or the absorption of other toxins into the blood may filter through the kidneys causing gene mutations and thus producing cancerous cells.

And then there's Non-Hodgkin's Lymphoma, also referred to as "NHL". This is a big name for a big disease. Non-Hodgkin's Lymphoma is a cancer that travels through the blood and primarily affects the body's lymph nodes. The lymph nodes are small structures that spread throughout the entire body. When the nodes are not infected, they would ordinarily help the body fight pollutants and disease. Because NHL travels through blood and can affect just about every lymph node, it's symptom may present themselves through an array of indicators. There may be chest pain, or difficulty breathing, or abdominal pain, or subtler signs like swollen lymph nodes, an annoying cough, fatigue or night sweats. There are no known causes for NHL, but characteristics that might increase one's risk are being over sixty years old, having used immunosuppressant drugs (these are drugs taken prior to an organ transplant), or toxins that have found their way to the blood stream.

The final cancer that I will mention is Thyroid Cancer. This cancer is usually, but not always, detected with a lump or a sizable swelling on the front of the neck. This kind of cancer will attack both men and women; however, women are three times more likely to be diagnosed with it. Other potential symptoms might include a pain that radiates from the neck to the ears, hoarseness, trouble swallowing or a continual cough. There are no defined causes of Thyroid Cancer, however research indicates that persons of Asian descent present a greater risk of this type of cancer.

Something to remember is that although I have mentioned several risk factors for different types of cancers, there are very few clear and absolute signs to look out for prior to a cancer diagnosis. It is important to see a doctor as soon as possible if you feel there is any cause for a health concern. Also note, that I've only mentioned a few, out of more than one hundred different types of cancer. In an attempt to be proactive, you should pay close attention to your body and its normal health patterns. If you recognize any differences, then I recommend that you to make an appointment and discuss the topic with a doctor.

TREATMENTS

Cancer treatment is not a one size fits all type of therapy. Specific treatments are based on the patient's age, other health conditions and how the patient responds to the treatment. Some people will have only one type of treatment while others may have several types of treatments and therapies. It can be confusing to understand exactly what each type of treatment is targeting, and what outcome can be expected, therefore, if the treatment or therapy is not explained by the doctor, make it a point to ask what are the benefits, risks and side effects that your loved one will experience.

The most common cancer treatments are:

- Surgery – which is an invasive operation where a surgeon cuts into the body and physically removes the cancerous tumor.
- Radiation Therapy – which is the process where a machine outside of the body directs high doses of radiation waves directly into the tumor.

- Chemotherapy – this is the process by which one or more very powerful cancer fighting drugs are administered either intravenously or in some cases by pill.

- Hormone Therapy – its purpose is to block hormone production in organs where cancer needs the hormones in order to grow. Hormone blockage can be done with pills, injections or surgery.

- Immunotherapy – this form of treatment stimulates the body's immune system to recognize cancer cells and destroy them. Several types of immunotherapy are used to treat cancer and can be administered intravenously, orally or with a topical solution.

- And the last one I'll mention is Stem Cell Transplant. This is when stem cells are donated from another person and transplanted into the cancer patient's bloodstream where they can help generate healthy new blood cells. This is typically done by blood transfusion.

These are only to name a few. Several other types of treatments exist but are not mentioned here. Therefore, any and all questions concerning therapeutic cancer treatments should be discussed with a healthcare provider for more clarity.

4. THE SUPPORT PERSON

Did someone ask you for help with their cancer journey, or did you volunteer? Or are you just thinking about volunteering for the position? I'm not going to sugarcoat this journey that you're considering or have already embarked upon; it's not an easy journey, nor is there much reward. So if you agreed to walk this path with your loved one, for any other reason than because you love them and you want to do what you can to ease their troubles, then you may experience your own difficulties. This is a journey that requires patience and compassion.

Who and what is a support person? Regardless of if you were asked, you volunteered, or you happen to be in a situation where it's expected for you to be the support person, then you are in the position of providing support and care for someone who is suffering with cancer. You are undoubtedly a friend, family member or someone the cancer patient trusts and believes they can lean on throughout this journey. You will conceivably be one of the most important persons in your cancer patient's life following their cancer diagnosis. You are the person who will be number one on the list of late night calls and texts when they can't sleep because they're scared and in need of positive or encouraging words. You are likely the person they will tell when they are nauseous and can't keep anything down, or when their hair starts to fall out, or their feet hurt, or they lose finger and toenails. You will be the one they call when they're depressed and feel like giving up. You will need to be mentally prepared to hear all of this and more because each of these instances will happen and because they are all stumbling blocks on the cancer journey.

If you've decided to take on this role, I'd like to share a few tips that were helpful to me as I accompanied my loved one through her cancer struggles. One thing to remember is that in this role, you don't have to be a healthcare worker, you just have to care about their health. This kind of care should be given willfully and with an open heart. When it becomes challenging, it may sometimes be necessary to take a step back and adjust your attitude by reminding yourself of why this person is important to you. There will be times that they don't need your assistance, or what they need will be something simple for you to achieve. However, it is quite possible that there will be times when the care required is overwhelming or exhausting. During any or all of these times, it will be less challenging and more helpful to you if you're in the right mindset before offering your assistance for a task.

COMMUNICATION

As with any good relationship, open communication is essential between the cancer patient and you as the major support person in order to become a cohesive team working towards the same goals. You, and your loved one, will want to be a trusting and solid team by always being on the same page. In order for your team to operate as efficiently as possible, consideration of both sides is necessary when organizing the upcoming tasks. You both deserve transparency of each other's expectations, feelings and the reality of what can or cannot be done. Transparency between the two of you will go a long way in establishing the trust that you are being considerate toward each other, and that both of your feelings and viewpoints are also being considered. This journey requires understanding and flexibility on both sides.

Instead of jumping in with the autopilot set on go, go, go, it may be helpful to have an initial conversation about expectations and the reality of the situation. This is mainly for you both to get on the same page with regards to the next steps and what's ahead. Both of you should you have the opportunity to express how you feel about the cancer journey. There's potentially a lot to discuss. However, you shouldn't get discouraged if your loved one doesn't have much to say initially. Remember that a cancer diagnosis could have a traumatic effect on the psyche and the patient might need time to come to grips with it. Most patients need time to incorporate how intensely this will affect their lives as they go forward. This diagnosis will affect them more personally than anyone else. When a cancer patient receives the news of their diagnosis, it may possibly have a devastating effect. They might possibly be overwhelmed and experience an array of emotions. The diagnosis may also produce thoughts of resentment, embarrassment, or maybe the idea that they'd prefer to handle matters alone. Therefore, a conversation about their health management may not happen right away, but they will likely open up at some point.

After hearing and digesting the fact of what's happening to their body, it's plausible that their first sentiments will be that of denial or fear. These can be separate emotions that may surface either together or independently and at different times. Denial may include a reaction of shock or disbelief. As a result, they may seem stunned and are unable to express their feelings. They may need time and patience to mentally work through the information they've been given. This is okay, but if at all possible, don't allow them to linger in denial for too long. It is imperative that they face the situation and determine how to they're going to handle it in order to promote the best outcome for their health.

Unfortunately, cancer doesn't wait for its victims to be ready, it aggressively continues to grow without permission. Fear, though related, is different than denial. Fear can produce feelings of hopelessness, confusion and being overwhelmed, which can individually or cumulatively be a gateway into depression. It is partially your job as their support person to help them cope with this conceptual chaos. I say partially your job, because you can only make suggestions on coping mechanisms, but it is ultimately up to them to make the mental adjustments.

BE POSITIVE

So how do you handle conversations and discussions with your loved one during one of the most distressing and painful times of their life? You encourage them through positive words and actions. Encouraging words should be the trend. It's best to refrain from contrary insinuations or undertones like, "you really don't have anything to complain about." This will not have a positive impact and may only make your loved one feel insecure. Instead of comments that could be misconstrued as criticism or demeaning, you can motivate them by placing emphasis on positive conditions. Encouragement is the key. Help them to practice acceptance of the moment and how to look for a silver lining in every situation.

Create small goals; the goals can be something as ordinary as keeping a doctor's appointment or remembering to take their medicines. Acknowledge the smallest of goals as an accomplishment. Consistently being grateful for the small things generally add up to a lot of little accomplishments, and this may lead to a positively accomplished day. It may also help to create an attitude of gratitude, which allows us to be mindful of our blessings. You should also exercise being a good listener. It's important that they know their concerns are being heard, but a response is not always necessary. There are often times that a patient doesn't want feedback or for you to help solve their problem, they might just need to vent their worries or apprehensions to someone who will listen.

DEALING WITH BAD ATTITUDES

It is not uncommon for people who are ill to frequently have bad attitudes, particularly if the illness is caused by a disease that can end in death. Unfortunately, the reality is that the face of some illnesses cannot always be transformed with a smile because the pain or frustration is just too great. As a support person, your job of caring for this special person may present its own set of challenges. But, if you change your perspective, and look at it from the patient's point of view, then you may understand that for them, this is not just challenging, but is possibly life threatening. They may see their greatest challenge through all of this is just in staying alive.

There may be times when cancer patients view their problems as being so intense and overwhelming, that they will lash out verbally and are unable to suppress their anger. We, as support people have no control over their reactions, but we can control how *we* respond to the negative words or actions that are mostly expressed out of frustration or exasperation.

Even if they can't smile through this difficult journey, you can. A gesture as simple as a smile can often times improve someone else's mood. Smiles are contagious, so there's always a chance that it'll rub off. But even if it doesn't rub off on your loved one, the upside is that there are still health benefits for you. A genuine smile can lead to a reduction in blood pressure, stress relief, or a balance of your own temperament.

You've heard of the saying, 'be the bigger person', now is the time to humble yourself to that guidance. If you can honor your commitment of helping your loved one throughout this process of healing, by being the 'bigger person' regardless of their good or bad words and actions, then you are being true to yourself and true to your commitment by respecting however they choose to deal with their struggles of this dreaded disease.

In the midst of perceived disrespect or rudeness, take a long, deep, breath and resist the impulse of returning emotional responses to their negativity or outbursts. Try to respond with kindness. If you respond negatively to rude or malicious comments, the negative exchange will only escalate and create hurt feeling on both sides, which can be damaging to the relationship and to you personally. On the other hand, kindness begets kindness. Although one should not give with the intentions to receive, showing compassion or speaking compassionate words is generally appreciated and tends to soften the intended receiver's mood, words and actions.

Cancer can be a very destructive disease. It can destroy one's ability to smile, to think clearly and to be hopeful. Cancer can take away any and all positive emotions and even a positive outlook. It can take away someone's joy. When one is faced with something so devastating it can threaten that spark that gives them life and it may become very hard for them to have a positive attitude and maintain a hopeful outlook. It is unwarranted but may be easy for that person to take their sorrow, anger and fear out on the person who is physically or emotionally closest to them at that time.

Releasing feelings of helplessness in a negative tone is part of being human. When taking care of and providing support to someone who is in a seemingly state of helplessness, it is important to understand where these emotions are coming from and the agony they are experiencing. This journey is not about you, so don't take every negative action personally. Their emotions, no matter how they're expressed, are about their ability or inability to live with their cancer diagnosis.

If it's at all possible, when negativity seems to be rearing its ugly head, take control of the conversation with an attempt to change the subject to something that's not such a sensitive issue. Changing the direction of the conversation allows you the chance to be proactive with the topics of discussion, instead of reactive to negative dialogue.

Bad attitudes, at times, lead to mean and hurtful words and actions. Mean and hurtful words and actions are commonly interpreted as abusive behaviors. It is never okay to let someone else willingly use offensive language or behave in a way that would cause you mental, physical or emotional anxiety or pain. Should this happen, it is completely within your right to remind them that their words or actions are insensitive and cruel.

No one likes to initiate confrontational discussions, but when your well-being is at jeopardy, it becomes a necessary evil. When having a discussion regarding a bad attitude or hurtful words and actions, try to refrain from using terms that would put them on the defense and possibly intensify their bad behavior. Take a moment, or a day, to consider exactly what you want to say and the best way to deliver your thoughts. If you choose not to speak about this verbally, a letter or text may be more preferable. Choose your words carefully but get your point across. Nonetheless, it may be helpful to anticipate and be prepared for both positive and negative outcomes.

Your loved one may or may not agree with you, they may or may not apologize and they may or may not think you're being spiteful or vindictive. Nevertheless, the confrontation allows the patient to reconsider, and hopefully understand how you feel about being the target of his or her aggressions. It also opens the space for the two of you to resolve conflicts. However, if you're dealing with someone who becomes increasingly belligerent or aggressive, it will become necessary to set boundaries on what's acceptable conduct when you're together. In the event that the situation becomes unbearable you may have to give notice that you will no longer be available if they cannot control their hostility.

If your loved one seems continually miserable and unhappy, it may be an early sign of depression. The word 'Depression' is not just a noun that refers to someone's unpleasant or overwhelmed mood, it is a clinical diagnosis of a true illness. If your loved one seems to have lost interest in normal activities that previously brought them joy, or if they are constantly irritable and lack emotional control, I would suggest that you ask their doctor or assigned social worker for recommendations on how to help them overcome their feelings. Treatment for depression may require medication or a therapy session here and there in order to get them feeling back to normal.

Fitting in therapy sessions may seem inconvenient on top of everything else you two are going through, but caring for their mental health is just as important as caring for their physical health. If office visits with a therapist, a counselor or a chaplain are not preferred, there are alternatives types of appointments such as telephone sessions, online sessions and even YouTube videos that can be watched. If your loved one is showing any signs of depression, don't ignore them or take the symptoms lightly because untreated depression can lead to more serious mental disorders further down the line.

5. DAILY - WEEKLY - MONTHLY

Everyone has good days and bad days, but this is even more true with cancer patients. Mental or physical uncertainty is basically the day to day status quo for both the cancer patient and their support person. This is undoubtedly a very scary and stressful time that will require your patience and flexibility. If you are the support person, you are the sidekick to the superhero. They have the hard job of battling cancer; your job is to manage everything else associated with it and within your control. This includes a wide range of objectives from attending doctor visits, or picking up medications to just listening while they vent, cry or laugh.

Being a support person will have its challenges. If you get frustrated, keep in mind the reason you chose to selflessly be of service. Let me remind you of one reason, because in spite of any and everything, this person holds a special place in your heart.

Other persons in your loved one's circle may also volunteer to be a support person. The more the merrier. There will certainly be enough tasks to pass around, though it's important that you all work together for the good of your loved one. These will be stressful times for everyone involved and your wellbeing and mental health are important too.

For this cancer journey, you, your loved, and anyone else that offers to help are a team. The team can consist of just you and your patient, or it can include several people who are willing to assist when help is needed. The team works together to lessen burnout by sharing information, and performing activities that aren't exclusive to the patient. And though it may seem insignificant, you should name your team. A team name reinforces the shared spirit and commitment dedicated to your loved one at this time.

Good communication is imperative. It would be helpful to have planning sessions to make plans for your team. The planning sessions can be done on a daily, weekly or monthly basis and will add organization to the current and future goals. This will ensure that the goals are met in a timely manner and completely achieved. Team planning is an activity that can be done face to face, by text messages or conference call. This time can also be a team bonding activity and a time that can be carved out to have coffee, lunch or simply visit with the team members and catch up on things happening outside of the cancer journey.

When making a plan for the week or month, I suggest that you first determine what you'd like to be the end result, then fill in the details regarding how you plan to get to the end result.

For instance, let's say your loved one has an appointment on Thursday at 3:00pm. The goal is to get them to the appointment and back home. You must decide how to get them there. Are you available? How long is the appointment expected to last? Will someone need to stay with them, or can they be dropped off? Will they need mobility assistance? Is a car or van necessary? Will there be parking fees?

Take time to journal or document your plan ideas because each event will likely require some degree of time and effort from you. Allow yourself to be flexible and to realize that the cancer journey is fluid and often requires modifications or adjustments to your initial plan, so don't get frustrated when things unexpectedly change. My advice is to simply practice going with the flow.

KEEP A SCHEDULE

The most effective way of planning for the upcoming days, weeks or even months is to list everything on a schedule. When you can visually see the task and appointments that lie ahead, it's a huge help with time management. Make sure you schedule the dates and times of everything cancer and non-cancer related that your loved one must participate in. This will include appointments such as primary doctor visits, oncology visits, seeing a specialist, laboratory visits for bloodwork, x-rays, treatments and even phone calls with a counselor or a social worker. It's a good idea to merge your personal or work agenda onto the same schedule so you can realistically see when you can and cannot be of assistance, and therefore plan accordingly.

There are several ways to maintain a schedule.

a. For those of you that are 'old school', a pen or pencil and a daily planner or monthly calendar would work just fine. If you don't already have a planner of some type, one can be purchased at almost any store that sells business type products, including Dollar and Ninety-Nine Stores.

b. For those of you who spend most of your day on a computer or tablet, most processing systems have a free planner or calendar. There are built in templates for Microsoft Word and Microsoft

Outlook. If you are an Apple user there is a MacOS calendar. If you use something other than a Microsoft or Apple product, search your system for a calendar option because one likely exists.

c. For those of us that that are never further than a breath away from our cell phones, there are several planning apps that can be downloaded, however the simplest and most cost effective route would be to simply use the calendar that is already installed on your phone. It's easy to detail and review any and all appointments on a daily, weekly or monthly basis.

By successfully scheduling all the cancer related events, it not only provides you with a way to accomplish small goals, and manage your time, but it is also a way to avoid scheduling conflicts while prioritizing what's most important for that particular time.

ACCOUNT FOR TRAVEL TIME

Cancer patients may have medical appointments weekly or even biweekly appointments. It's vital for them to attend each one of the appointments. There may be occurrences when several appointments may be scheduled at different medical facilities during the same week, or once-in-a-while even the same day. It may be valuable for you to be included when setting up or arranging the appointments with each medical provider.

This way, you can ensure that the appointments are sufficiently spread out and won't overtax the patient, you or the team. It may be difficult to juggle everything that needs to be done, but remember that the primary objective of cancer appointments and treatments is to cure or delay advancement of the disease.

Trying to accompany your patient to each and every appointment can be an exhausting undertaking; this is why it's important to have team involvement when making out the schedules. With each appointment you must consider how your patient will get there and back. Doctor appointments may take an hour or two, whereas chemotherapy may take four or more hours, and a radiation treatment may mean an all day visit or even a short hospital stay.

Make sure you are prepared for how much time each appointment will take. Some doctors prefer to schedule their appointment, bloodwork and radiation or chemotherapy all in one day; this may be easiest on the patient, but difficult to fit into your personal agenda. Therefore, it may be to your advantage to call in advance and get a general idea of how long each procedure may take. If it's perceived to be a long appointment or therapy visit, you may decide to drop off your loved one and make arrangements to either return at a selected time, or have someone else pick up the patient at a designated time and location.

You may want to accompany your loved one to the doctor and therapy visits to provide them with moral support, but because of your own commitments, it may not be practicable for you to attend each and every visit. In these types of situations, you could use the support of another person or teammate with dropping off, picking up or attending the visits when you cannot. However, if no one else is available to assist with the visits, there are companies that you can contact and arrange for them to provide transportation assistance for your cancer patient. You can contact the American Cancer Society or even use an internet search engine to find businesses in your area that provide free or discounted transportation for cancer patients. If your loved one has a wheelchair or mobility issues, this is something to consider when choosing the appropriate form of transportation.

Something else to consider is that cancer will not go away on its own, therefore if it is impossible for your loved one to attend a scheduled appointment, you should reschedule the appointment at the earliest convenience to continue prevention of further spread of the disease.

MEDICATION

Some cancer medications are given in the hospital or clinic, and other medications are prescribed to take at home. Medications can be dispensed in an assortment of ways. Most prescribed medications come in the form of pills or liquids, yet other forms might include injections or topical solutions. No matter what form of medication is prescribed, it is imperative that the directions are followed. The bottle or container should be checked for the patient's name, the name of the medication, the amount, frequency and time of day it should be taken. These checks should be made each time the medication is taken or put into a pill box. Almost all prescribed medications come with printed instructions. However, there may be instances of office or telephone appointments where a doctor will give verbal instructions on how and when to take a medication. In the event that the instructions are given verbally, you should write them down and keep them in a secure place.

Your loved one may have pill bottles that have different names and label instructions, but most of the prescription containers will look alike. It may be helpful if you provide a method of organization on when and how the dosages should be administered. We found that putting the medications in a weekly pill box worked for us. We then created a medication schedule which allowed us to keep track of the days and times each drug was to be taken. A pill box is a rectangular container, used to separate and organize when medications should be taken.

There are a variety of pill boxes that may span over three days, seven days or even a twenty-one-day time period. Most pill boxes have multiple compartments that are divided by the days of the week and some may be further expanded to include morning, noon and evening divisions.

When considering your loved one's medication, you also need to consider that there might be suggested supplemental or over-the-counter medications in addition to what was prescribed by the doctor. There may also be medications that the patient was already taking prior to the cancer diagnosis. Almost always, a patient's prescribed and supplemental medications will be noted during the initial health history and an assessment of their interactions will be made at that time.

If additional non-prescribed supplements are considered along the cancer journey, they should first be approved by the doctor. All medications, prescribed or not, should be included in the pill boxes and on the medication schedule. If all medications and supplements are approved as 'safe to take' by the doctor, then it is also safe to store them together in the pill boxes by suggested day and time.

Filling pill boxes can be tedious, but using them is much more efficient than taking the meds directly from their containers. By assisting in keeping the medications organized, whether it seems appreciated or not, just know that you are also doing your part to help in their healing process.

Your involvement is also helping to control their physical discomfort and even the condition of your loved one's body and peace of mind.

6. THEIR PERSONAL NEEDS

In addition to making schedules, attending hospital visits and managing medications, there are personal needs your loved one will also have. This is another consideration you will need to plan for. Cancer therapies and treatments are not a 'one size fits all' remedy and will differ depending on the type of cancer. One patient may experience mild side effects that will not affect their daily routine, while another person may have severe and overwhelming side effects that are completely unbearable. In either situation, they may need your assistance following treatments.

Consider also that cancer is not only a shock to the physical body, but also a mental shock. Therefore, your love and care as their support person shouldn't end with the business side of cancer, you should also be there for the more personal situations or even moral support. Their personal needs may start with getting them through the side effects.

DEALING WITH SIDE EFFECTS

A diagnosis of cancer, and cancer treatments, have been known to have physical, emotional and spiritual side effects on the patient. Side effects are the unintended consequences of the illness and treatments, including physical therapy or even drug therapy. No side effects are exactly the same for cancer patients and will vary depending on the type of cancer and the subsequent treatment.

Physical side effects may include mild inflictions such as fatigue, dry mouth, diarrhea or constipation, loss of appetite, bruising or problems sleeping. However, many patients suffer from much graver effects like incontinence, infections, hair loss, hypothyroidism, lung issues, skin problems or temporary memory loss. There are also occasions where side effects develop into lifelong problems leaving the patient to deal with diabetes, eye cataracts, heart issues, hearing loss, infertility, organ damage, osteoporosis, or neuropathy (which is basically nerve damage).

Unfortunately, I have only mentioned a few of the physical side effect. There are numerous resulting effects of cancer or cancer treatment, and I emphasize again, it's different for every patient. Be sensitive to whatever your loved one says they are feeling during this journey or after a specific treatment. One person may have a chemotherapy treatment and be able to go to work afterwards, while another patient may have the same type of chemotherapy treatment and vomit profusely afterwards. Though there are common side effects associated with cancer treatment, there is no way to absolutely predict which side effects your loved one may fall prey to. My advice is to simply be sensitive and supportive of whatever they say they're experiencing.

Cancer has a way of also taking a serious emotional toll on its sufferers. Along with everything else, many cancer patients experience side effects in the form of various stages of depression, anxiety or more severe mental health issues. Don't take it personal if your loved one has abrupt mood swings, or suddenly lashes out, or spends more time crying.

It's during these times that you should know and remember that the disease prompts unexpected behavior. Calmly remind yourself and your loved one that you are there to help. Most oncology centers have social workers to help patients and their families navigate through the cancer journey. If you have a deep concern about the emotional well-being of your loved one, do not hesitate to reach out to the social worker in your network to ask for help. You might want to also express your concerns if you have any.

Another side effect of cancer may be the spiritual distress your loved one might experience. Spirituality means different things to different people. For some, it's religion or a connection to a higher power, for others it's a connection to nature or the environment, and then there are those that see and respect their body as a temple. No matter what beliefs are held, a cancer diagnosis may shake that belief and the patient may question their faith. Spirituality is an individual path that fails or grows within a single person, especially during a time of crisis.

If your loved one's faith is waning, they may feel abandoned or rejected by what they've once held in great esteem and this too could lead to depression. It may help to point out the blessings that still remain in their life. Encourage them to find and feel the peace in their hearts or either make time to heal their wounded heart. You can suggest that they keep a daily gratitude journal. If they can write down at least three things they are grateful for on a daily basis, then this would be a step toward a more positive mood.

PERSONAL AND SPECIAL WAYS TO HELP

Cancer is alive and comparable to a parasite feeding on your body. Living with, and trying to survive cancer can be incredibly difficult. It's a challenge that requires all the strength your loved one can give. Cancer and the aggressiveness of its treatments will likely suck most of life's energy from your loved one's mind, body and soul. It's not just another disease, it's a disease that targets the body's healthy cells and destroys them, leaving its victims feeling depleted or extremely fatigued and often in agonizing pain.

If you have struggled with something that's left you feeling utterly worn-out and unable to talk yourself into pushing forward, then you know how they will feel on most days -- they do not want to do much of anything. Having you there to do the pushing for them would be a relief. It will be helpful if you could organize a way for them to have their household needs taken care of, and give them the opportunity to focus on their recovery. Here are a few suggestions to consider and possibly schedule with your team;

- Prepare meals or snacks that can be readily available because their appetite will come and go. This is especially important if they live alone. Be sure to consult them on any dietary restrictions.

- Do their grocery shopping.

- Wash their laundry.

- Change their bed linens.

- Set out comfortable apparel or clothing easy to get into.

- Make sure magazines, books or the TV remote are easily accessible.

- Mail or send their bills.

Most cancer patients experience some degree of neuropathy. This is a weakness or numbness in the hands and feet caused by the disease. It's quite plausible that they can have varying degrees of neuropathy, from tingling and numbness in their hands and feet to having little feeling or no use of them. This is one of the reasons your loved one may require assistance with their personal or household needs. Their personal needs might include things like brushing their hair, getting dressed or ready for the day, keeping their nails cut and trimmed, massaging their extremities or applying lotion to their skin.

THOUGHTFUL THINGS

Arranging to give your time and attention to your loved one during these difficult times is a huge gift and a testament to how much you love and care for them. Nothing more is required other than for you to be in the present when you're with them. However, from time to time you may realize that there are a few minor items that could be useful during their cancer journey and make things a little easier for the both of you. What seems like simple little extras that may not cost much by themselves such as lotions, powders, clippers, a foot massager, headache medicine or protein shakes; but after making several trips to the store to pick up this item or that item, the costs can eventually add up.

Some of the small personal items may seem to be only for personal pleasure, but may be what exactly what's need for boosting their morale. If you have the extra money or don't mind paying for high end merchandise to help give them comfort, then by all means, shop until you drop. However, if money is an object of concern don't fret, some form of the extra but necessary needs, can also be found at a ninety-nine cents or dollar store.

FINANCES

Unfortunately, the cancer journey is an expensive journey and most people have challenges trying to manage the costs. Many people don't want to ask their doctors about the price of treatments and medications because they don't want the expenses to change their quality of care. Nevertheless, it's critical to help your loved one be aware of the financial obligations, so they are prepared to deal with them. Otherwise, this will be one more thing to stress over.

You can help them to deal with their financial responsibilities by making a financial plan. Include in your plan as many cancer related expenses as you can think of. Common expenses are the co-pays for hospital or clinic visits, treatments, and unexpected purchases like wigs, light apparel or specific foods.

If your patient is fortunate enough to have some form of health insurance that covers cancer and cancer related treatments, this will be a blessing because it will pay for a lot of the expense. Still, the out-of-pocket expenses can be financially crippling. The good news is that there are several programs and resources that offer assistance with cancer related expenses.

Following the diagnosis, your loved one should be assigned a caseworker, social worker or financial counselor. If they haven't been assigned one, be sure to ask the doctor to refer one. The financial counselor should be able to explain what to expect financially, and guide your loved one on how to make payment arrangements, or direct them to cancer financial aid programs and resources. The financial counselor or the social worker can also help with suggestions on home health agencies, medical equipment and even hospice.

Another option for finding help with finances is to search the internet. There are a number of websites that detail options for cancer related expenses. There are also websites that specifically focus on cancer concerns such as the National Cancer Institute, the Center for Disease Control and the American Cancer Society, which all share links for financial resources and assistance.

Additionally, if your loved one has a church membership or frequents a particular church, they or you can reach out to the church ministry for prayers and help in the form of financial support. Many churches have a network of ways to care for their congregation and community.

7. TAKE CARE OF YOU

Properly caring for your loved on their cancer journey is of utmost importance, but it does not come above taking care of yourself. A support person can sometimes get so wrapped up in caring for the cancer patient that they begin to lose sight of their own personal goals and objectives. If this happens it can become very stressful and have an overwhelming negative effect on your emotional wellbeing, as well as your individual experiences and relationships. The last thing you want to do is to become so consumed in your loved one's journey that you detach from your own life. This kind of detachment could lead to your own feelings of resentment and depression.

As critical as your loved one's needs may seem, you should always put your well-being first. You cannot effectively care for someone else if you're not in a mentally and physically healthy place yourself. A number of resources will tell you that in order to establish and maintain balance in your life and have healthy relationships with others, you must first be happy and feel good about yourself. Requiring time for personal self-care is not being selfish, it is respectfully granting yourself a 'time-out' so that you can replenish your energy, grace and joy.

There are ample ways to practice self-care, it all depends on your particular preferences and likes. However, because I consider this to be the most significant aspect of being a support person, I have a number of suggestions for you:

- Music – who doesn't love some form of music to relax and get lost in? No matter if you decide to simply sit back and tap your foot, or get up and breakout some dance moves, the vibes of good music is always good for the soul.

- Carve Out Some Daily Downtime – this would be a time in your day or evening that you set aside some time just for you. You can work on a hobby, exercise, engage in a television show, or do some other mindless activity like a candlelit bath with your favorite drink. This is your time to take care of you.

- Meditate – humbly put… take the time to just breath, clear your mind and think of happy thoughts or how grateful you are to just be right here, right now.

- Recite Affirmations – these are words or phrases that you'd routinely repeat to create a positive mood or attitude. You can either find an affirmation that's already published in a book, or on the internet, or on an app, or make up your own. It doesn't matter where you get it, only that it makes you feel good.

- Create your own support team – make time to talk with friends, relatives or church members about topics not related to cancer.

- Laugh – make it a point to watch a comedy or listen to a comedian on a podcast, YouTube or any other streaming source in an effort to lift your mood and lessen the stress.

- Declutter – when you declutter your home, car or personal surroundings, on some level it also releases the clutter in your mind. This opens up mental space that can be filled with positive energy and happiness.

- Eat Well – healthy eating is good for your overall mental and physical well-being. It reduces the risks of depression and protects against certain illnesses. A balanced diet can also reduce stress and the risk of heart attack or stroke.

- Sleep – getting enough sleep is essential to life. It allows your mind and body the chance to recharge and get energized for the next round of activities.

When our lives become intimately entwined in someone else's life, as is often the case with caregivers, there's a possibility that we'd provide wonderful care for them, but completely neglect ourselves. Be good to yourself. Preserve the right for self-respect and self-compassion, because the better we take care of ourselves, the better we can take care of others.

8. FINAL COMMENTS

A person diagnosed with stage one cancer can experience as much anxiety as a person diagnosed with stage four cancer. Cancer can have a life altering impact on the mind, body and soul. Try to remember that this is a critical time in their life, and the effort it takes to heal from cancer can be a time of crisis for any patient. You, as their support person, will probably be the most important person in their life during their journey. There is a lot to be done. There will be months of hospital and therapy appointments. It may be physically or mentally taxing to keep up with everything, even with the sufficient scheduling of doctor visits, medications and other miscellaneous tasks.

In time, you'll have to watch the physical changes of their body breaking down and experience their emotional ups and downs, all while possibly dealing with their sudden negative outlook or attitude. For some of you, it will feel like an emotional roller coaster; and through it all you'll need to keep your composure and be compassionate. Two important things to remember are: be kind to them and be kind to yourself.

You might be the most loving and caring support person on this earth, but you will still need to set boundaries. You must maintain a healthy balance between taking care of your loved one, and taking care of yourself. I would advise that you to let your family, friends and employer know of your commitment to the cancer journey with your loved one. This way, your family and friends may be understanding of why you're away from home more often or why you're more tired when you are home. Also, your employer may be able to add more flexibility to your schedule.

Finally, hold onto a positive image of what life will look like for each of you once you get to the end of the cancer journey, and work towards getting there. However, until you reach the end, remember to exhale between tasks, say your affirmations and be strong enough to help them fight the disease. Your strength will give them the courage to get through the battle. You can do this!

ACKNOWLEDGEMENTS

Thank you to my readers for taking the time to read this book. It was written to serve as a suggestive guidebook for those who are searching for a kind and loving way to care for someone with cancer. I hope it has been helpful, and you are successful on your journey with your loved one.

I would also like to thank my family for their assistance in creating this book. First to my husband Johnny, who offered only love and patience as I sat in a corner chair for so many days and nights. Thank you for never complaining about the long hours I'd spend in front of a computer instead of in your loving presence. Thank you to my three children, Julian, Tiffani and Timerri who keep me encouraged and uplifted. They always reach for the stars, so how can I do any less. Thank you to my mom Phyllis, who has always been my biggest motivator and also my biggest cheerleader. I thank you from the depth of my heart for your personal and professional contributions to this book. And finally, thank you to Cynthia, Cindy and all of my friends who have inspired this book, both in sickness and in health.

THE END

Made in the USA
Middletown, DE
25 September 2023

39327920R00036